This Book

BELONGS TO

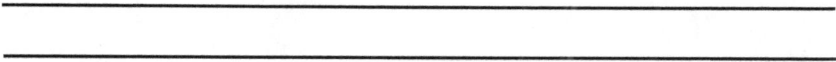

Dedication

This Health Journal is dedicated to all the people out there who want to keep track of their health and document their findings in the process.

You are my inspiration for producing books and I'm honored to be a part of keeping all of your Health notes and records organized.

This journal notebook will help you record your details about tracking your health.

Thoughtfully put together with these sections to record: Family History, Surgery Record, Dental, Check-ups, Wellness, Medication, Appointments, Diet & Exercise, Meal Tracker, & Exercise Tracker.

How to Use this Book

The purpose of this book is to keep all of your Health notes all in one place. It will help keep you organized.

This Health Journal will allow you to accurately document every detail about your health. It's a great way to chart your course through recording everything about your health.

Here are examples of the prompts for you to fill in and write about your experience in this book:

1. Personal Information
2. Insurance Contact
3. Medical Contact
4. Family Medical History
5. Surgery Record
6. Dental
7. Medical Check Up
8. Monthly Wellness
9. Monthly Medication
10. Monthly Appointments
11. Monthly Diet & Exercise Plan
12. Monthly Meal Tracker
13. Monthly Exercise Tracker

PERSONAL INFORMATION

Contact Details

Name:

Email:

Phone:

Address:

Emergency Contacts:

My Physician/GP Details:

INSURANCE CONTACT

List

Name   **Agent Name**

Insurance Type   **Policy No.**

Contact   **Cost**

Notes

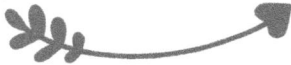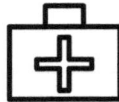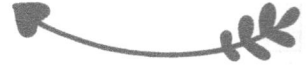

Name   **Agent Name**

Insurance Type   **Policy No.**

Contact   **Cost**

Notes

MEDICAL CONTACT

List

Name
Speciality

Phone No.
Email

Address

Notes

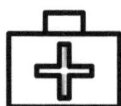

Name
Speciality

Phone No.
Email

Address

Notes

MEDICAL CONTACT

List

Name	Speciality

Phone No.	Email

Address	

Notes

 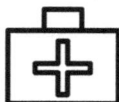 

Name	Speciality

Phone No.	Email

Address	

Notes

MEDICAL CONTACT

List

Name   **Speciality**

Phone No.   **Email**

Address

Notes

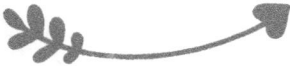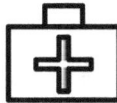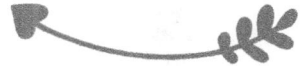

Name   **Speciality**

Phone No.   **Email**

Address

Notes

MEDICAL CONTACT
List

Name	Speciality

Phone No.	Email

Address

Notes

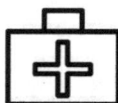

Name	Speciality

Phone No.	Email

Address

Notes

FAMILY MEDICAL HISTORY

List

Name   **Relation**

_____

Disease

_____

Allergies/Illness/Other

_____

Notes

_____

_____

 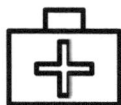 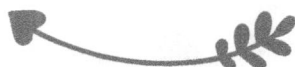

Name   **Relation**

_____

Disease

_____

Allergies/Illness/Other

_____

Notes

_____

_____

FAMILY MEDICAL HISTORY

List

Name

Relation

Disease

Allergies/Illness/Other

Notes

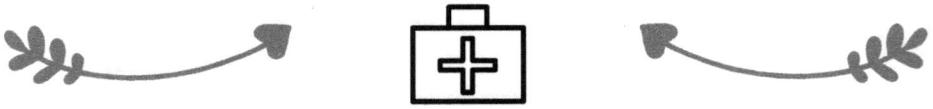

Name

Relation

Disease

Allergies/Illness/Other

Notes

FAMILY MEDICAL HISTORY

List

Name   Relation

Disease

Allergies/Illness/Other

Notes

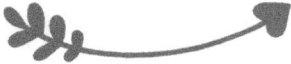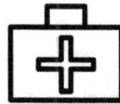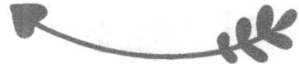

Name   Relation

Disease

Allergies/Illness/Other

Notes

FAMILY MEDICAL HISTORY
List

Name

Relation

Disease

Allergies/Illness/Other

Notes

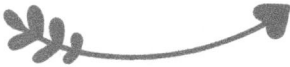 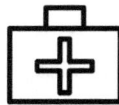 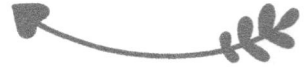

Name

Relation

Disease

Allergies/Illness/Other

Notes

SURGERY RECORD

List

Surgery   **Doctor**

Date   **Release Date**

Complications

Notes

_____

_____

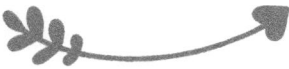 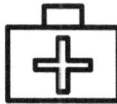 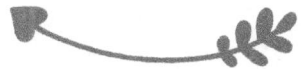

Surgery   **Doctor**

Date   **Release Date**

Complications

Notes

_____

_____

SURGERY RECORD

List

Surgery   **Doctor**

Date   **Release Date**

Complications

Notes

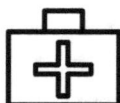

Surgery   **Doctor**

Date   **Release Date**

Complications

Notes

DENTAL CHECK UP

List

Dentist

Date

Next Appointment

Contact Details

Notes

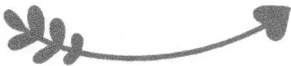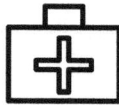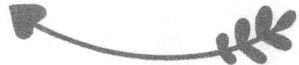

Dentist

Date

Next Appointment

Contact Details

Notes

DENTAL CHECK UP
List

Dentist

Date   **Next Appointment**

Contact Details

Notes

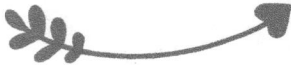 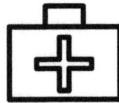 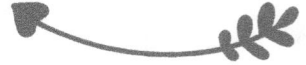

Dentist

Date   **Next Appointment**

Contact Details

Notes

DENTAL CHECK UP
List

Dentist

_____

Date   **Next Appointment**

_____

Contact Details

_____

Notes

_____

_____

 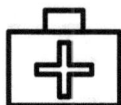 

Dentist

_____

Date   **Next Appointment**

_____

Contact Details

_____

Notes

_____

_____

DENTAL CHECK UP
List

Dentist

Date   **Next Appointment**

Contact Details

Notes

_____

_____

 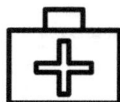 

Dentist

Date   **Next Appointment**

Contact Details

Notes

_____

_____

MEDICAL CHECK UP
List

Doctor   **Hospital**

Date

Treatment/Diagnosis

Notes

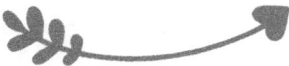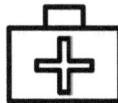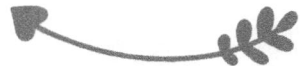

Doctor   **Hospital**

Date

Treatment/Diagnosis

Notes

MEDICAL CHECK UP

List

Doctor   Hospital

Date

Treatment/Diagnosis

Notes

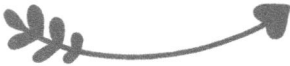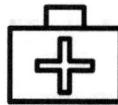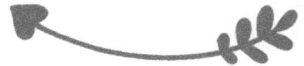

Doctor   Hospital

Date

Treatment/Diagnosis

Notes

MEDICAL CHECK UP

List

Doctor   Hospital

Date

Treatment/Diagnosis

Notes

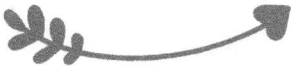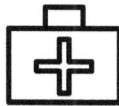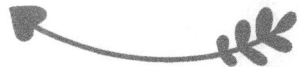

Doctor   Hospital

Date

Treatment/Diagnosis

Notes

MEDICAL CHECK UP

List

Doctor   Hospital

Date

Treatment/Diagnosis

Notes

_____

_____

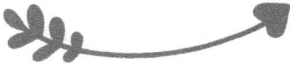 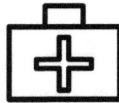 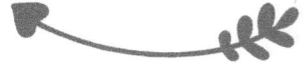

Doctor   Hospital

Date

Treatment/Diagnosis

Notes

_____

_____

MEDICAL CHECK UP

List

Doctor   Hospital

Date

Treatment/Diagnosis

Notes

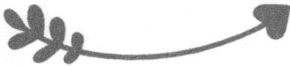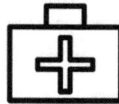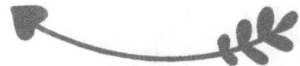

Doctor   Hospital

Date

Treatment/Diagnosis

Notes

MEDICAL CHECK UP

List

Doctor   Hospital

Date

Treatment/Diagnosis

Notes

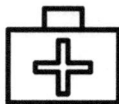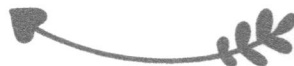

Doctor   Hospital

Date

Treatment/Diagnosis

Notes

JANUARY

MY MONTHLY WELLNESS
Tracker

Mon	Tue	Wed	Thu	Fri	Sat	Sun

Notes

MY MONTHLY MEDICINE
Tracker

Mon	Tue	Wed	Thu	Fri	Sat	Sun

Notes

MY MONTHLY APPOINTMENT
Tracker

Mon	Tue	Wed	Thu	Fri	Sat	Sun

Notes

MY MONTHLY DIET & EXERCISE
Plan

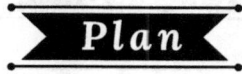

My Weight:

Workout Dates:

Diet Plan:

Weight Loss Goal:

Fitness Classes:

Notes:

MY MONTHLY MEAL

Mon	Tue	Wed	Thu	Fri	Sat	Sun

Notes

MY MONTHLY EXERCISE

Tracker

Mon	Tue	Wed	Thu	Fri	Sat	Sun

Notes

FEBRUARY

MY MONTHLY WELLNESS
Tracker

Mon	Tue	Wed	Thu	Fri	Sat	Sun

Notes

MY MONTHLY MEDICINE
Tracker

Mon	Tue	Wed	Thu	Fri	Sat	Sun

Notes

MY MONTHLY APPOINTMENT
Tracker

Mon	Tue	Wed	Thu	Fri	Sat	Sun

Notes

MY MONTHLY DIET & EXERCISE

Plan

My Weight:

Workout Dates:

Diet Plan:

Weight Loss Goal:

Fitness Classes:

Notes:

MY MONTHLY MEAL

Tracker

Mon	Tue	Wed	Thu	Fri	Sat	Sun

Notes

MY MONTHLY EXERCISE
Tracker

Mon	Tue	Wed	Thu	Fri	Sat	Sun

Notes

MARCH

MY MONTHLY WELLNESS
Tracker

Mon	Tue	Wed	Thu	Fri	Sat	Sun

Notes

MY MONTHLY MEDICINE
Tracker

Mon	Tue	Wed	Thu	Fri	Sat	Sun

Notes

MY MONTHLY APPOINTMENT

Tracker

Mon	Tue	Wed	Thu	Fri	Sat	Sun

Notes

MY MONTHLY DIET & EXERCISE

Plan

My Weight:

Workout Dates:

Diet Plan:

Weight Loss Goal:

Fitness Classes:

Notes:

MY MONTHLY MEAL

Tracker

Mon	Tue	Wed	Thu	Fri	Sat	Sun

Notes

MY MONTHLY EXERCISE

Tracker

Mon	Tue	Wed	Thu	Fri	Sat	Sun

Notes

APRIL

MY MONTHLY WELLNESS
Tracker

Mon	Tue	Wed	Thu	Fri	Sat	Sun

Notes

MY MONTHLY MEDICINE
Tracker

Mon	Tue	Wed	Thu	Fri	Sat	Sun

Notes

MY MONTHLY APPOINTMENT
Tracker

Mon	Tue	Wed	Thu	Fri	Sat	Sun

Notes

MY MONTHLY DIET & EXERCISE
Plan

My Weight:

Workout Dates:

Diet Plan:

Weight Loss Goal:

Fitness Classes:

Notes:

MY MONTHLY MEAL

Tracker

Mon	Tue	Wed	Thu	Fri	Sat	Sun

Notes

MY MONTHLY EXERCISE

Tracker

Mon	Tue	Wed	Thu	Fri	Sat	Sun

Notes

MAY

MY MONTHLY WELLNESS
Tracker

Mon	Tue	Wed	Thu	Fri	Sat	Sun

Notes

MY MONTHLY MEDICINE
Tracker

Mon	Tue	Wed	Thu	Fri	Sat	Sun

Notes

MY MONTHLY APPOINTMENT
Tracker

Mon	Tue	Wed	Thu	Fri	Sat	Sun

Notes

MY MONTHLY DIET & EXERCISE

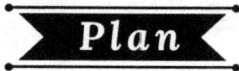

Plan

My Weight:

Workout Dates:

Diet Plan:

Weight Loss Goal:

Fitness Classes:

Notes:

MY MONTHLY MEAL
Tracker

Mon	Tue	Wed	Thu	Fri	Sat	Sun

Notes

MY MONTHLY EXERCISE
Tracker

Mon	Tue	Wed	Thu	Fri	Sat	Sun

Notes

JUNE

MY MONTHLY WELLNESS
Tracker

Mon	Tue	Wed	Thu	Fri	Sat	Sun

Notes

MY MONTHLY MEDICINE
Tracker

Mon	Tue	Wed	Thu	Fri	Sat	Sun

Notes

MY MONTHLY APPOINTMENT
Tracker

Mon	Tue	Wed	Thu	Fri	Sat	Sun

Notes

MY MONTHLY DIET & EXERCISE
Plan

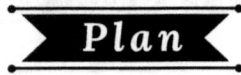

My Weight:

Workout Dates:

Diet Plan:

Weight Loss Goal:

Fitness Classes:

Notes:

MY MONTHLY MEAL
Tracker

Mon	Tue	Wed	Thu	Fri	Sat	Sun

Notes

MY MONTHLY EXERCISE
Tracker

Mon	Tue	Wed	Thu	Fri	Sat	Sun

Notes

JULY

MY MONTHLY WELLNESS
Tracker

Mon	Tue	Wed	Thu	Fri	Sat	Sun

Notes

MY MONTHLY MEDICINE
Tracker

Mon	Tue	Wed	Thu	Fri	Sat	Sun

Notes

MY MONTHLY APPOINTMENT
Tracker

Mon	Tue	Wed	Thu	Fri	Sat	Sun

Notes

MY MONTHLY DIET & EXERCISE

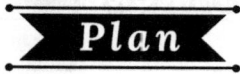

Plan

My Weight:

Workout Dates:

Diet Plan:

Weight Loss Goal:

Fitness Classes:

Notes:

MY MONTHLY MEAL

Tracker

Mon	Tue	Wed	Thu	Fri	Sat	Sun

Notes

MY MONTHLY EXERCISE

Tracker

Mon	Tue	Wed	Thu	Fri	Sat	Sun

Notes

AUGUST

MY MONTHLY WELLNESS

Tracker

Mon	Tue	Wed	Thu	Fri	Sat	Sun

Notes

MY MONTHLY MEDICINE
Tracker

Mon	Tue	Wed	Thu	Fri	Sat	Sun

Notes

MY MONTHLY APPOINTMENT
Tracker

Mon	Tue	Wed	Thu	Fri	Sat	Sun

Notes

MY MONTHLY DIET & EXERCISE
Plan

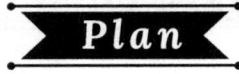

My Weight:

Workout Dates:

Diet Plan:

Weight Loss Goal:

Fitness Classes:

Notes:

MY MONTHLY MEAL

Tracker

Mon	Tue	Wed	Thu	Fri	Sat	Sun

Notes

MY MONTHLY EXERCISE
Tracker

Mon	Tue	Wed	Thu	Fri	Sat	Sun

Notes

SEPTEMBER

MY MONTHLY WELLNESS
Tracker

Mon	Tue	Wed	Thu	Fri	Sat	Sun

Notes

MY MONTHLY MEDICINE
Tracker

Mon	Tue	Wed	Thu	Fri	Sat	Sun

Notes

MY MONTHLY APPOINTMENT
Tracker

Mon	Tue	Wed	Thu	Fri	Sat	Sun

Notes

MY MONTHLY DIET & EXERCISE
Plan

My Weight:

Workout Dates:

Diet Plan:

Weight Loss Goal:

Fitness Classes:

Notes:

MY MONTHLY MEAL
Tracker

Mon	Tue	Wed	Thu	Fri	Sat	Sun

Notes

MY MONTHLY EXERCISE
Tracker

Mon	Tue	Wed	Thu	Fri	Sat	Sun

Notes

OCTOBER

MY MONTHLY WELLNESS
Tracker

Mon	Tue	Wed	Thu	Fri	Sat	Sun

Notes

MY MONTHLY MEDICINE
Tracker

Mon	Tue	Wed	Thu	Fri	Sat	Sun

Notes

MY MONTHLY APPOINTMENT
Tracker

Mon	Tue	Wed	Thu	Fri	Sat	Sun

Notes

MY MONTHLY DIET & EXERCISE
Plan

My Weight:

Workout Dates:

Diet Plan:

Weight Loss Goal:

Fitness Classes:

Notes:

MY MONTHLY MEAL
Tracker

Mon	Tue	Wed	Thu	Fri	Sat	Sun

Notes

MY MONTHLY EXERCISE
Tracker

Mon	Tue	Wed	Thu	Fri	Sat	Sun

Notes

NOVEMBER

MY MONTHLY WELLNESS
Tracker

Mon	Tue	Wed	Thu	Fri	Sat	Sun

Notes

MY MONTHLY MEDICINE
Tracker

Mon	Tue	Wed	Thu	Fri	Sat	Sun

Notes

MY MONTHLY APPOINTMENT
Tracker

Mon	Tue	Wed	Thu	Fri	Sat	Sun

Notes

MY MONTHLY DIET & EXERCISE

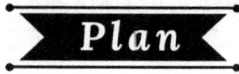

Plan

My Weight:

Workout Dates:

Diet Plan:

Weight Loss Goal:

Fitness Classes:

Notes:

MY MONTHLY MEAL

Tracker

Mon	Tue	Wed	Thu	Fri	Sat	Sun

Notes

MY MONTHLY EXERCISE
Tracker

Mon	Tue	Wed	Thu	Fri	Sat	Sun

Notes

DECEMBER

MY MONTHLY WELLNESS
Tracker

Mon	Tue	Wed	Thu	Fri	Sat	Sun

Notes

MY MONTHLY MEDICINE
Tracker

Mon	Tue	Wed	Thu	Fri	Sat	Sun

Notes

MY MONTHLY APPOINTMENT
Tracker

Mon	Tue	Wed	Thu	Fri	Sat	Sun

Notes

MY MONTHLY DIET & EXERCISE
Plan

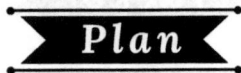

My Weight:

Workout Dates:

Diet Plan:

Weight Loss Goal:

Fitness Classes:

Notes:

MY MONTHLY MEAL
Tracker

Mon	Tue	Wed	Thu	Fri	Sat	Sun

Notes

MY MONTHLY EXERCISE
Tracker

Mon	Tue	Wed	Thu	Fri	Sat	Sun

Notes

www.ingramcontent.com/pod-product-compliance
Lightning Source LLC
Chambersburg PA
CBHW051030030426
42336CB00015B/2802